grown-up
&
gorgeous

in your 60s

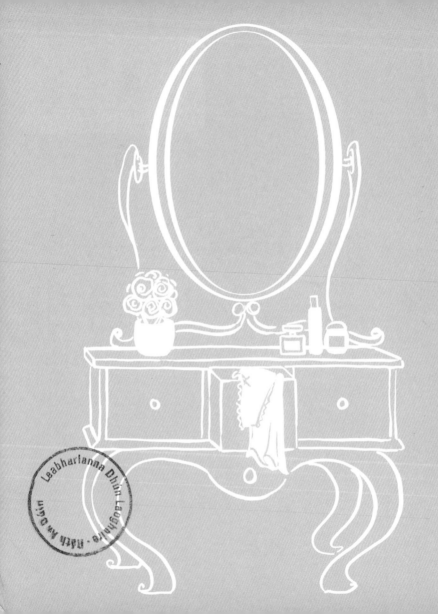

grown-up & gorgeous

in your 60s

Pamela Robson

EBURY
PRESS

Acknowledgements: Dr Mary Dingley, President of the Australasian Society of Cosmetic Physicians; Tanja Mrnjaus, ID Couture, Melbourne, Sydney and Brisbane; Dr Shane Rea, Barshop Institute for Longevity and Aging Studies, University of Texas; Ken Gordon & Toni Adams, Musculo-Skeletal Clinic, Spring Hill, Queensland; Dr Cathy Gaulton, Pacific Cosmetic Surgery, Brisbane, Queensland; Jean Hailes Foundation; Wellesley College Biology Department, Maryland; American Academy of Peridontology

Contents

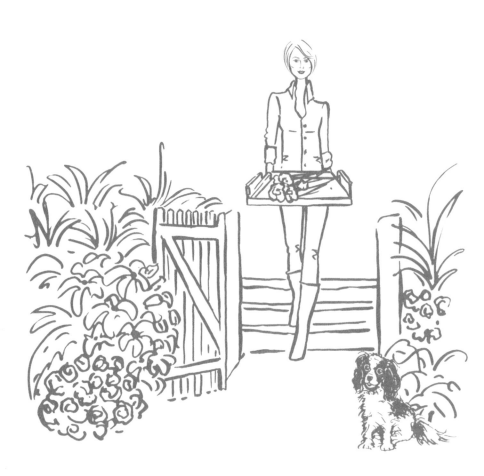

*T*here's never been a better time to be in your 60s. You've had enough experience to know who you are and what you want out of life. It was your generation who pioneered the women's movement, embraced the Pill and fought for equal pay. Then, you redefined what it meant to be a woman – now you are redefining what it means to be 60. While you might be keen to give the 9 to 5 the flick, you're not ready to spend the rest of your life pottering. Instead, you'll work part-time or run a business from home; you'll volunteer and travel. There have never been so many choices, and so many things to do. You want to look healthy and attractive, be mentally alert and physically active, and stay relevant to the community we live in. You don't want to become Germaine Greer's 'invisible woman', with one sensibly shod foot in the grave. This book is to help you make the most of it all. Welcome to your 60s!

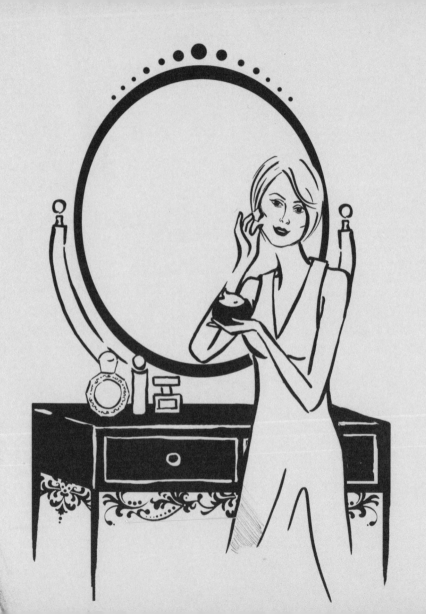

Beauty

*T*oday, it seems, everyone wants to look younger than they are. But most of us aren't trying to kid ourselves that we can pass for our daughters. We want to radiate inner health, vitality – basically, look as good as we can for our age, while still looking like *ourselves*. Beauty is far more than skincare, make-up and a great haircut – yet these things can go a long way to boosting your confidence. And caring about your appearance is a sign you value yourself. Yes, it's time for some 'me' time!

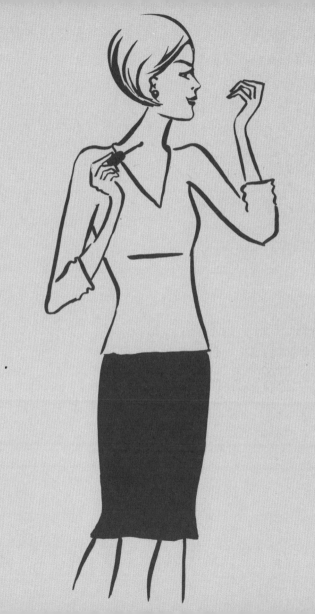

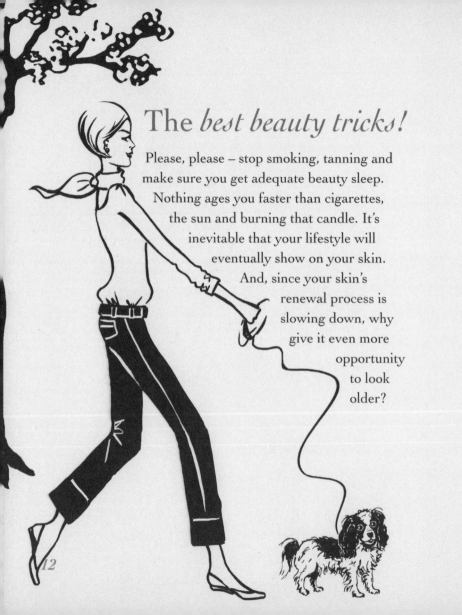

The *best beauty tricks!*

Please, please – stop smoking, tanning and make sure you get adequate beauty sleep. Nothing ages you faster than cigarettes, the sun and burning that candle. It's inevitable that your lifestyle will eventually show on your skin. And, since your skin's renewal process is slowing down, why give it even more opportunity to look older?

The skin you're in

If you think that your skin is 60, you'd be wrong. It's actually about 30 days old. In fact, your whole body has probably just celebrated its 15th birthday. That's the time it's taken to rebuild itself from top to bottom. According to the latest scientific research, every cell in your body is continually being replaced by a new one. This new way of looking at life has enormous implications for the way we age in the future.

Skincare

You're unlikely to be experiencing breakouts, but you will be battling dryness, wrinkles and dullness – and your skin may be feeling significantly thinner. Less is best, here. You don't want to irritate your skin with harsh cleansers, or dry things out further with abrasive scrubs.

Skincare basics

Cleansing, exfoliating and moisturising, day and night, will keep your skin looking fresh and dewy. As mentioned above, choose products that are as gentle as possible – there's no need for expensive, complicated formulas. Continue using sunscreen (moisturisers that contain SPF are handy), and certainly start using skin protection if you haven't already done so – it's never too late. Also, a good dermatologist or cosmetic doctor will be able to advise you on how best to care for your skin – now, and for future decades.

Beautiful extras

As well as your basic skincare routine, these three
additions will work wonders:

Eye cream: The skin around your eyes is more delicate
than the rest of your face. Try a lightweight eye
cream that absorbs well into your skin and leaves it
smooth. Apply it in gentle dabs and wait a while before
applying make-up.

Face serums: These concentrated liquids are packed
with skin-nourishing nutrients that help to prevent
visible signs of ageing. Apply after cleansing and before
moisturising.

Face oils: These old-fashioned beauty products work
beautifully on dry skin – look for ones containing sweet
almond, olive, avocado and jojoba oils, and massage
them gently over your skin whenever it feels in need of
extra hydration.

A brief skin lesson

It helps to know exactly what you're caring for.

Epidermis – the outer layer: The cells of this outer
layer are constantly being sloughed off as new cells
rise from deeper in the skin to take their place.
Exfoliation – scrubs, peels, Intense Pulsed Light, laser
– removes these outer cells, and speeds up skin renewal
by stimulating cell changeover. It revs up collagen
production, too. The epidermis also holds the cells that
produce skin pigment. The condition of your epidermis
determines how 'fresh' your skin looks and also how
well your skin absorbs and holds moisture. As we age,
the outer cells become stiff and the skin can't hold
moisture the way it used to.

Dermis – the middle layer: This is the thickest of the skin layers, made up of a tight, strong matrix of collagen and elastin fibres, bathed in hyaluronic acid. Collagen provides structural support and elastin makes the skin more elastic. Hyaluronic acid retains water like a sponge, absorbing more than 1000 times its weight. It helps to attract and hold water around the collagen and elastin, moisturising the skin and plumping it up. As we age, cell renewal slows and we produce less collagen, elastin and hyaluronic acid, so the dermis becomes thinner and less elastic – meaning wrinkles will form.

Subcutaneous layer – the fat cells: Underneath the dermis is the subcutaneous tissue, consisting mainly of fat cells, which helps support your face structure. The loss of this tissue, which happens with age, means that things will start to sag.

Confused about face creams?

One of the best ways to make your skin look dewy and plump is to use moisturisers. The cosmetic industry is massive and the sheer volume of creams on the market can be very confusing. It's important to know a couple of things about them before you buy. Because wrinkles develop deep in the dermis, face creams can't work to remove or stop them. Generally speaking, a face cream can't penetrate the top layer of your skin. What they do well is retain (not add) moisture on your skin's surface.

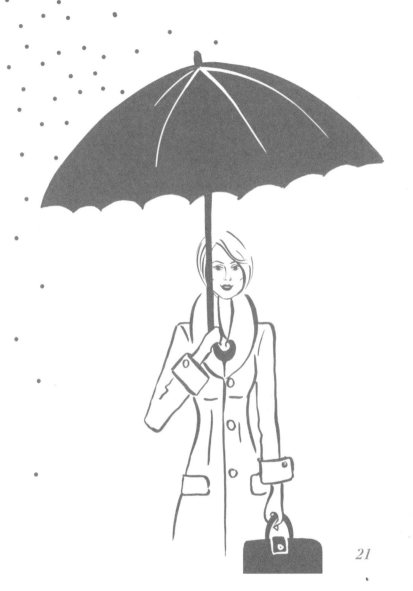

21

Hyaluronic acid

Most face creams can only act as a protective barrier to stop your skin from drying out. There are, however, some newer topical hyaluronic creams and gels available from dermatologists and cosmetic doctors that can add more moisture. The hyaluronic acid acts like a sponge to absorb and hold moisture.

Tretinoin (Retrieve or Retin A)

This prescription-only cream has been around for more than 30 years as an acne preparation. About a decade ago its abilities were recognised in smoothing skin and softening lines and wrinkles. Derived from vitamin A, it is the only topical product that has been shown to change the structure of the skin. Basically, being slightly acidic, it removes the outer layer of the skin, encouraging faster cell turnover. You must use it sparingly (otherwise it can irritate), and avoid the sun.

Vitamin C

Our skin is made up of about 75 per cent collagen, and, as we age (especially post-menopause), our bodies become less efficient at making it. Vitamin C is the key player in the formation of collagen. Like other topical face creams, most vitamin creams are really only moisturisers. A couple of vitamin C creams, however, are known to produce good results.

Can-do creams

Yes, your mother was right – you are what you eat. A big research project by Melbourne's Monash University studied 450 people aged 70 or over to see if there was a link between how wrinkly they were and what they ate. They found that those who ate mainly vegetables, fish, low-fat milk products and tea were the least wrinkled. They concluded that the magic ingredients for protecting against wrinkles were vitamin C, calcium, phosphorus, magnesium, iron and zinc. People with the most wrinkles tucked into full-fat foods such as butter, margarine, cheese, red meat, soft drinks, cakes and pastries.

It's what's on the inside . . .

The good skin diet

You don't need a scientific study to tell you that the best way to stay looking youthful is to eat a diet full of fresh fruit and vegies, good fats (avocado, olive oil, nuts, salmon), and to drink plenty of plain old water. Cut back on skin-drying caffeine and alcohol, and cell-damaging sugar.

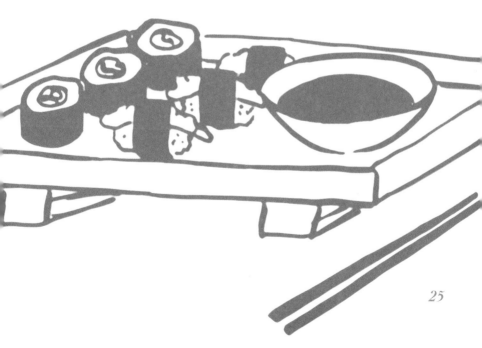

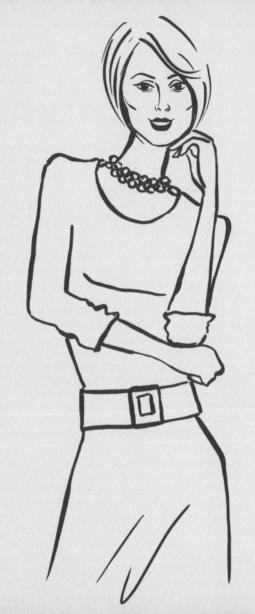

Make-up

The older we get the more we seem to be tempted
to increase the amount of make-up we wear, when we
should be lightening up. As we age we should strive all
the more to look natural. Being painted can look cute
on a 20-year-old, but as our skin texture roughens and
wrinkles, lines and folds develop, thick make-up is not
a good look. The natural look – in make-up, hair and
the clothes we wear – looks confident and relaxed,
but most of all, healthy. And as we all know,
healthy = youth = beauty.

Natural doesn't mean going nude . . .

On the contrary, it means smart make-up – new technology has given us the option of using natural-looking products with light-reflecting, lifting and firming agents.

New-generation bases: A heavy powdery face in broad daylight is not a good look at any age. There are plenty of the advanced tinted moisturisers or lightweight foundations around, and many have lifting properties for mature skins.

Natural fake tans: Even in these sun-conscious days, a light golden tan can look radiantly healthy. While you are at the beauty counter, try a light bronzer with a translucent finish.

Creamy formulas: Cream blush is much easier to apply than the old powder varieties. Just smile and place a dot of creamy colour right on the rounded part of your cheek and blend it up towards the hairline using your fingertips. This will give you a lovely healthy glow. But make sure you blend it in well.

INSTANT PICK-ME-UPS

Here are five simple ways to have you looking
and feeling fresh.

Hydrate: *Plump skin by layering on a hydrating face cream
and a face balm (for extra-dry areas), dabbing on eye cream
and slicking on lip gloss. You'll look so dewy.*

Brighten: *Lighten the under-eye area with concealer – apply it as
close to the lower lashes and inner eye corner as you can, blending well.*

Glow: *Apply a pop of blush to the apples of your cheeks.*

Define: *Line your eyes and extend the line ever so slightly
beyond the outer corner of your eye.*

Shine: *After applying lipstick, add a slick of clear
light-reflecting, shimmering gloss over the top.*

The eyes have it

It's no wonder you're confused: your 60s often herald a loss of eye definition, and so you'd like to redefine their shape and colour with make-up – but the issue of crepey skin surely means that's a no-no? Not necessarily. Certainly it's a good idea to steer clear of powdery, shimmery, coloured or too-creamy eyeshadows (they'll simply settle in the creases and look clownish), but experts recommend a very light etching of soft eye pencil along your upper and lower lashline, along with mascara on the upper lashes (on the bottom lashes, it can emphasise dark circles). Avoid harsh black, especially if your hair and brows are silvery; choose brown, taupe and grey instead.

Update your look
instantly

Consider having your brows and lashes professionally tinted. It's relatively cheap, instantly creates definition, and is a great time-saving device. A good beautician or beauty therapist will be able to recommend the appropriate shade to suit your skin and hair colour.

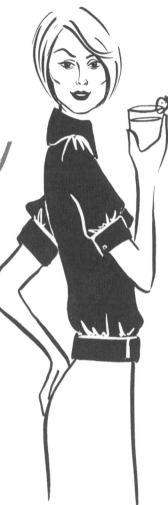

Ditch the dark, matte lippie . . .

. . . in favour of a luscious glossy pink. Dark colours make things look thinner, so it stands to reason that dark lipstick will do the same, and matte formulas can be very drying. Be careful with long-lasting lipsticks. By their very nature they have to be dry to stay put for longer. Do your homework: some of the newer long-lasters using advanced technology are far less drying. They usually come as a dual kit with a base and a gloss.

EXPERT TIP

Keep an old toothbrush handy to lightly exfoliate your lips. Apply a little balm or Vaseline to your lips, then gently buff off dry skin.

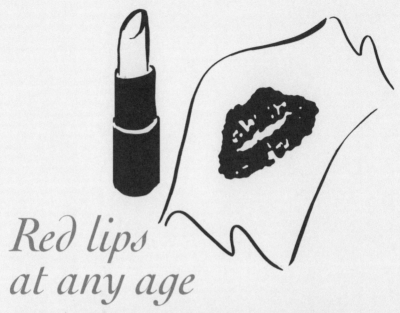

Red lips at any age

You *absolutely* must go easy on your eyes and blush when your lips are a standout colour. But, paired with a little black mascara, your red lips will be the epitome of chic. Coat your lips with liner before applying lippie to prevent bleeding of the colour into the lines around your mouth (it'll also help your lipstick last longer).

Sexy golden skin

A tan gives you the glow of youth and health. It masks a multitude of problems such as broken capillaries, stretch marks and cellulite. A tan also gives your body definition and can even help you look slimmer. And, since we all know not to sunbake, it's handy that the *safe* sun-kissed look now comes in a bottle. The beauty industry has invested a lot of money in developing a whole new generation of fake-tanners, so there's no need to be wary of pungent scents or orange streaks.

Want to DIY?

You can choose from mousses, sprays, creams and gels. They are genuinely easy to use and often come packaged with exfoliants to remove dry skin and moisturisers to smooth things over before the tan. If you aren't feeling confident, try the new body moisturisers that contain a light fake tan – you simply apply the body cream daily and the colour builds up naturally over time. This is also the easiest way to apply fake tan to your face – many of the biggest beauty brands have face moisturisers that also contain a light fake tan that builds up gradually, plus SPF, *plus* a tint for an instant glow. Amazing!

Prefer the pro touch?

For a special occasion, or to start your tan off, it's a good idea to have a professional in-salon treatment. This way you'll get a natural, streak-free, all-over colour. Most products dry within five or 10 minutes and you can go straight back to your daily routine.

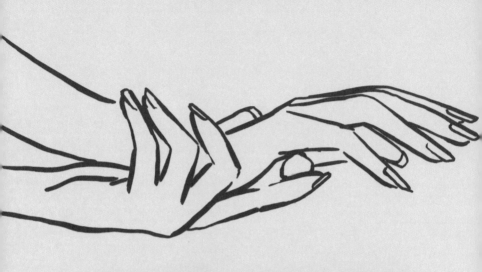

EXPERT TIP

Keep your hands and feet soft and supple, and your nails healthy, by soaking them in olive oil occasionally – it's a celebrity beauty secret.

Speed dial

These are the beauty professionals you
should have in your little black book.

Cosmetic doctor

Dermatologist

Brow stylist

Hair stylist

Beauty therapist

Cosmetic dentist

Hair

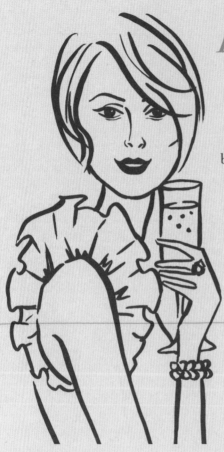

Since the tight perm and blue rinse is, thankfully, a thing of the past, your hair *can* be your crowning glory, your best accessory, and a shining example of style and health. Forget 'rules' about not being able to have long hair after a certain stage, or feeling like you must cover greys: as long as your hair is in good condition and is cut well, anything goes. It's all about what works with your lifestyle and hair type.

HAIR FACTS

★ Each person has about two million hairs; only about 100,000 are on your head.

★ Each hair follicle can grow many hairs over a lifetime: on average, each grows a new hair about 20 times.

★ A hair grows at a rate of about 1 centimetre a month.

★ The hair has a three- to six-year growth cycle.

★ The hairs don't grow in unison. They are out of sync with each other. If they grew together at the same rate we'd temporarily go bald from time to time. This is why, if you have laser hair removal, you need to go back to have the dormant hair treated.

★ The length that you can grow your hair depends on your genes. In some people, the hair falls out when it reaches the shoulders.

Keep it moving

There's nothing more ageing than a stiff hairstyle. These days, hair should be soft, casual, tousled. Above all, it needs to look natural and healthy. So put away the lacquer and talk to your hairdresser (they'll become your best friend once you find one that really understands you) about a style that is *easy* to maintain.

To colour or not to colour?

It's not only men who can be silver foxes. Well-cared-for grey hair can be stunning (use colour-correcting shampoo – your hairdresser can advise on this). If it's not for you just yet, enlist the help of a clever colourist at your hair salon. The older you get, the lighter you need to go. There is nothing so ageing as severe dark colour.

Update your look instantly

When grey roots start peeking through, make-up artists swear by this little trick: a dusting of dense powder eyeshadow (one matching your hair colour) will do a decent job of covering roots for the day.

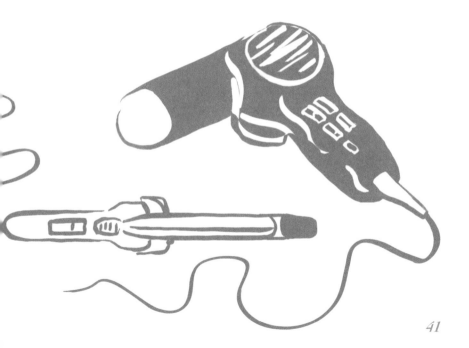

Things that can affect hair growth

* Stress

* Hormonal changes such as menopause

* Crash diets and alcoholism

* Poor general health and nutrition

* It is known that zinc plays a part in hair growth as does vitamin B, which also improves elasticity, strength and gloss.

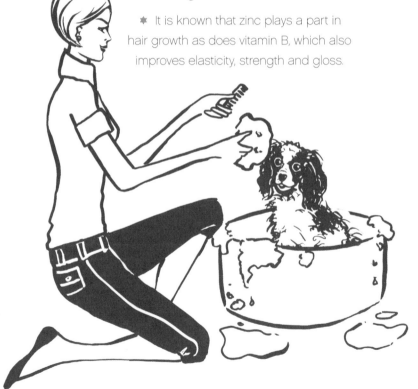

HAIR AS YOU AGE

The hair cycle becomes shorter, the follicles gradually stop producing long, strong hair, and the hairs become thinner and shorter.

About 5 per cent of middle-aged women have unwanted facial hair.

After menopause, the face becomes hairier, while the rest of the body's hair is slowly lost.

About 10 per cent of 65-year-old women have noticeable chin hair.

Thinning on top?

It's not only men who are self-conscious about thinning hair. For many post-menopausal women it can be a hugely sensitive issue. About 25 per cent of women between 50 and 60 experience hair loss, and it runs in families. But it's not just an age or genetic thing. It can be the result of illness, or even of too-tight hairstyles. Most of all, it can result from stress. If your hair is thinning, a good place to start is your doctor. They can help diagnose the cause and refer you to a specialist if necessary. You may be a candidate for hair-transplant surgery. This is an expensive procedure but it really does work. The doctor takes hair follicles from areas where hair is thicker and transplants them to areas where there are few. Sometimes the doctor will opt for a combination of surgery and medication, which helps promote regrowth. The results are now very natural.

Camouflage options

Your hairdresser can be a miracle worker, as the right cut (often involving layers), can make sparse hair look much thicker. And if you've got the face for it, get a short cut. It can look très chic. Just look at Maggie Tabberer – she's learned to deal with very fine hair by making the sleek style her statement look. Well-placed highlights, volumising shampoos and thickening styling products are also great options.

In your 60s, cosmetic procedures are less about preventative techniques (such as Botox) and more about filling and resurfacing. Of course, Botox still has its place (to help create a non-surgical brow-lift, for example), but the buzzwords for you are face sculpting, skin smoothing and non-surgical facelifts. One last word on Botox: if you're going to take this path, remember that less is more. You can always go back for further treatments, but too much too soon will leave you looking very unnatural.

There's no need to resort to the invasive facelifts of old. The cosmetic technology just keeps on getting better.

Non-surgical facelifts

Thermage: A non-surgical procedure that uses radio-frequency to tone skin. Heat created by the frequency causes the collagen to tighten. It's good for lifting jowls, upper eyes and brows (but it works best on people with little loss of elasticity to begin with). You'll need once-monthly treatments over several months to see results.

Titan: A new entry in the laser light therapy category, it heats the dermis which makes the collagen contract and tighten, and encourages the growth of new collagen. It's not a quick fix – you'll need treatments over about six months for results.

Acupuncture facial: Hair-thin needles are inserted into certain points on the face and scalp, and the needles make the underlying muscles contract or relax. You'll need quite a few treatments to see results.

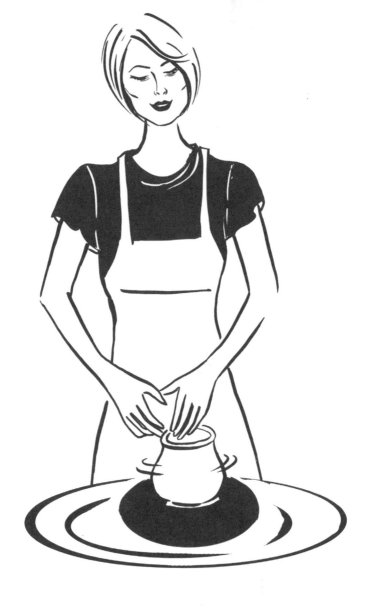

Face sculpting

One of the most exciting new directions for cosmetic medicine is facial sculpture. This is where synthetic fillers are used to plump areas of the face, either directly or by stimulating the skin and soft tissue to rebuild itself.

Hyaluronic fillers: These are injected to help define the jaw or build up cheekbones (the effect can last for a year or two). These fillers are also used to address hollows under the eye, which can occur as the cheek fat pad drops. They are also being used just under the eyebrow to help lift the upper lid and reduce drooping.

Sculptra: This synthetic acid stimulates the body to produce its own collagen. Used for facial sculpting, it can be injected into any area that needs volume. It requires a short series of treatments and lasts for about three years.

Skin smoothing

Smooth skin is equated with youth, so it's no wonder it's the Holy Grail of beauty. There is a battalion of cutting-edge technologies to help improve your complexion, each with its own area of specialty. They all try to match the skin rejuvenation properties of the original lasers, but without the long recovery period and the complications (such as permanent loss of skin pigment). Most are endeavouring to do this by reaching the lower levels of the skin while leaving the surface intact. How well these techniques work depends on how well your skin can make new cells. Your dermatologist or cosmetic doctor can advise you on the results you can expect.

IPL (Intense Pulsed Light): Dubbed the 'lunchtime treatment' (because you can go back to work after having it done), this is ideal for someone who wants a light 'polish' and to get rid of blotchiness. It's good for removing freckles, broken capillaries and liver spots. IPL is offered by medical practices and beauty salons, and it's quite gentle compared with the other options. A series of treatments is usually recommended, spaced at weekly intervals.

Fraxel laser: This treats the skin in a pixel fashion, creating hundreds of tiny wounds on a little bit of skin at a time; it triggers the body's healing process, speeding up the production of collagen and cells. Fraxel is excellent for treating acne scars and is the first technology to make a difference to stretch marks. It can also be used on the neck, chest and arms – areas considered more difficult to rejuvenate than the face. Generally, a series of treatments is required.

Plasma resurfacing: And we all thought plasma was for TVs . . . This resurfacing device converts a stream of nitrogen into gas, which is fired at the skin to remove the surface. Again, it aims to match the effectiveness of the old lasers without the side effects and long recovery times. Resurfacing is usually a one-off procedure.

Most skin resurfacing and tightening treatments are only performed by dermatologists and cosmetic doctors, however some treatments (such as IPL and light peels) are offered by beauty therapists. All of these treatments can burn, so it is important that you do your homework and find a practitioner who comes recommended, and who you know you can trust. President of the Cosmetic Physicians Society of Australasia, Dr Mary Dingley, suggests finding a practitioner who has both training and expertise in the specific procedure you're interested in. CPSA members specialise in cosmetic medicine, so patients can rest assured they are being treated by an appropriately trained and experienced practitioner.

Choosing your doctor

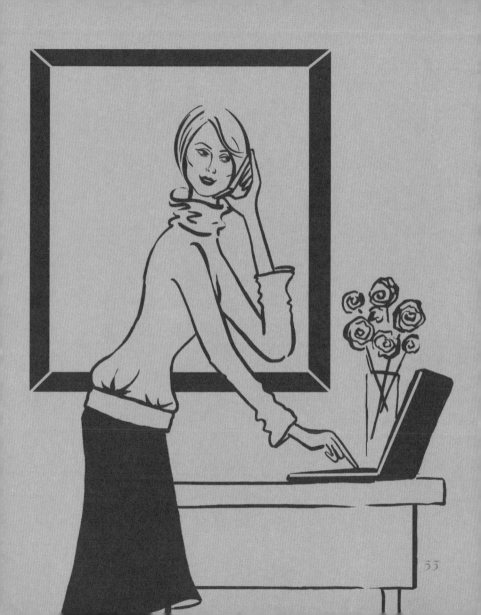

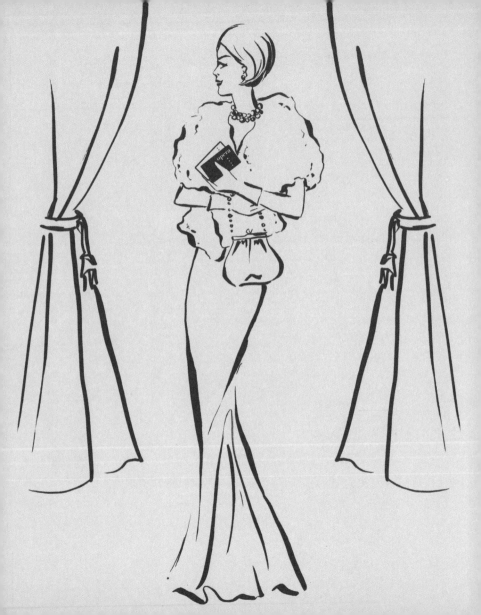

Wardrobe

When it comes to style, age matters less these days. The message from the professional stylists is: dress for your personality or lifestyle – not your years. The idea is to mix and match and add accessories to create a look that presents your individuality to the world. If this sounds daunting, it absolutely needn't be. Almost anything goes – as long as it doesn't look too contrived or too crazy. Don't be scared by fashion. It's meant to be fun.

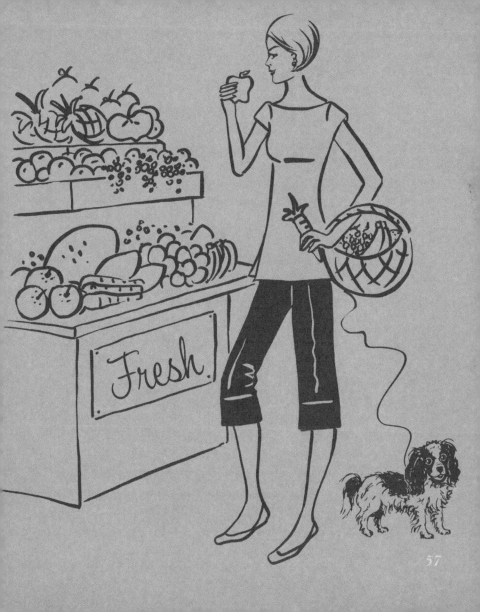

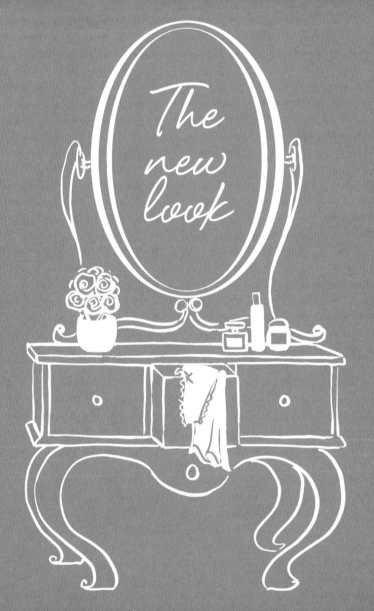

The
new
look

In the past, buying clothes was fairly straightforward. Every season, the designers told us what to wear; something was either 'in' or it was 'out' – and certain outfits were worn in certain situations. Today, jeans and T-shirts are worn to the office and the opera; silky cocktail dresses come out to play during the day. The turnover of trends is mind-bogglingly high. It's not surprising that many women just wash their hands of the whole thing, and stick to what they've been wearing for years.

The new rules

Today, about the worst thing you can do is to have everything matching. The contrived air hostess look of the 1960s is about as uncool as you can go – unless you are 16 and wearing it for its retro value. These days, the idea is to look effortlessly chic, as if you haven't tried too hard. Make this your mantra: casual is contemporary; contemporary is young.

Looks to avoid

The *Anne of Green Gables* look:
puffed sleeves and Liberty prints

★

The country & western singer look: short
fringed skirts and cowboy boots

★

The Miss Marple look: sensible shoes,
tweeds and twin-sets

★

The rock chick look: black leather jackets
and too-tight jeans

★

The 'I made it myself' look: strange colours
and fabrics with seams that stubbornly
don't quite match up

The classics

* A casual pair of jeans, and a pair for dressier occasions

* A trench coat in a neutral colour

* A black wool jacket

* A cashmere cardigan in a pastel or neutral colour

* Cotton tops (tees, singlets, long-sleeved tops) in classic colours

* A white shirt

* A simple black or navy knee-length skirt

* A neat little black dress

* Black tailored pants

* White tennis shoes

* Black pumps and black flats

It can save you money. Professional stylists are big in the UK and US and it's getting that way here in Australia. You'll find them under Image Consultants in the Yellow Pages. They've become part of the outsourcing trend and are brought in to help by women who haven't the time (or talent) to shop. Stylists also work with groups of women on shopping sprees. A session with a stylist can be a great gift idea for your next birthday, or 'just because'. If you spend your life thinking about others, this is the perfect antidote because it's all about *you*.

Get professional help!

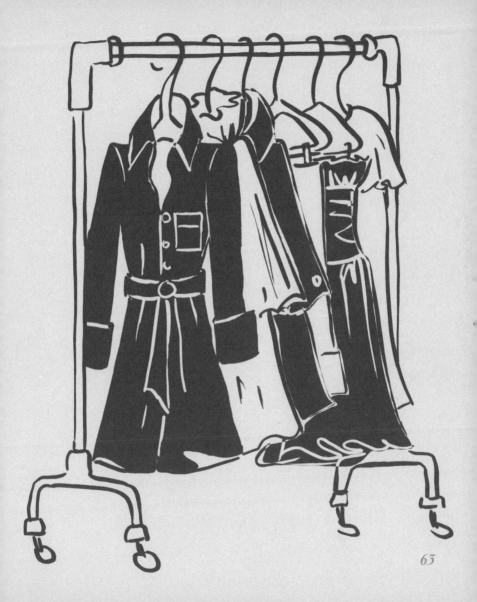

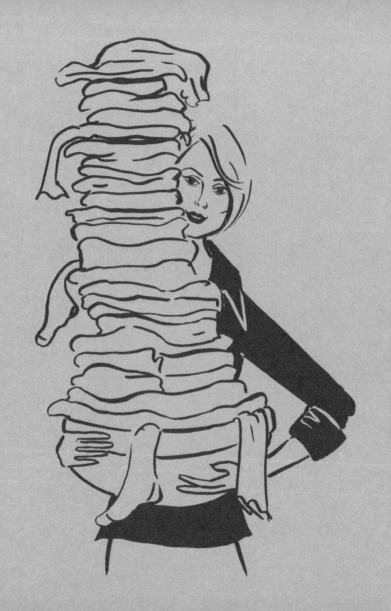

Clear the *clutter*

You can hire people to do this for you now. But, it's a good habit to get into yourself – and what better time to start!

Choose a time when you're feeling positive and decisive, and divide your wardrobe into three piles: things to throw away (items in need of major alteration, damaged pieces, 'skinny' clothes you'll never slim into), things to store for later (classic yet seasonal clothes), and things you wear all the time.

Consider your lifestyle, and what clothes are appropriate. If you no longer work, why would you want six business suits? If you hate the beach, why all those old swimmers? The idea (if you're ruthless enough) is that you end up with excellent basics, which you will revitalise with fresh pieces.

Budget!

This is an exciting time – the chance to freshen up your look. But there's no need to max out the credit card: chain-stores copy the catwalk so quickly these days that there's a look to suit every budget. Importantly, to make a budget work you must resist the impulse buy. Consider the 'gaps' in your wardrobe (perhaps you need a good trench coat, or a flattering pair of jeans) and make a list of items you will need. Do your research: spend a couple of weekends browsing and trying things on before you buy. If you feel the need for retail therapy, get it out of your system with accessories: belts and scarves are reasonably inexpensive, yet are a quick way to update your look.

HINT: DO YOUR HOMEWORK

Find style inspiration in celebrity role models; look at magazines; check out the designer collections on the internet; watch the fashion network on cable TV . . .

If there's a designer or store that you know can deliver the styles that suit you, do continue to buy from them. You aren't expected to become a different person! But don't get stuck in a fashion time warp.

Be loyal to your favourites

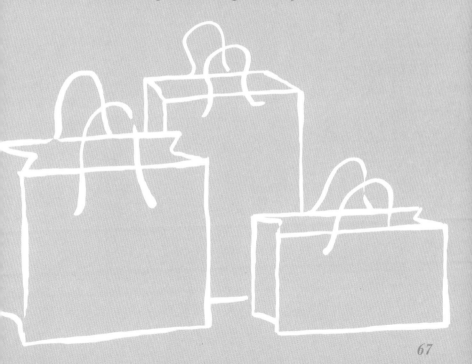

BOOB-BOOS

There's nothing worse than a light-coloured T-shirt worn
over a lacy (heaven forbid, black) bra.

★

Take care with the moulded cups. If you're flat-chested,
they're a boon, but if you have any chest at all, you can
look like a Wagnerian soprano at full tilt.

★

Too-small bras – the overflow can make you look
like you've got two sets of boobs.

★

Going bra-less in flimsy clothing. There's a time
when we can no longer let it all hang loose in public.
Now is that time.

Non-negotiable: a good bra (or five)

If there ever was an investment piece, the bra is it. The wrong one is unflattering, unhealthy and makes your clothes hang incorrectly. If you're wearing a bra that gives no lift and your boobs are just hanging around casually, you haven't a hope of looking stylish! Head straight to the lingerie section in a department store, get fitted by a professional and you'll wonder why on earth you didn't do it sooner. According to the experts, most women are wandering around in bras that are completely the wrong size and style – having a professional cast her objective eye over your assets can result in you wearing a completely different cup size, and can totally change the look of your boobs (for the better).

The bras you need

First, you'll need a T-shirt bra or two (it gives a smooth, natural, nipple-free silhouette) for everyday wear. Next, pick a good-quality sports bra (even if you don't jog, there are always more active occasions when you'll need the support). Finally, select a couple of pretty bras in printed cottons, and a sexy push-up number. Voila!

Whether you're still working or not, your wardrobe can be packed full of deliciously stylish casual wear (note the emphasis is on 'stylish'). The lynchpin of the casual wardrobe is the T-shirt. This little item is deceptive. It's fairly cheap to buy, so we regard it as being just one step up from underwear. Yet the right one can make a world of difference. Ideally, you'll have one in white, one in black and another in flattering grey marle. These days, good-quality black or white tees can be worn to dinner with sparkling jewellery, with jeans and bright coloured beads to a barbecue, or under a jacket for a business meeting.

The basic T-shirt

What suits you?

Pick a T-shirt with a little bit of Lycra so it's not too 'boxy' and starched, so it slightly hugs your shape. If your arms aren't what they used to be, make sure the sleeves hit mid-bicep (avoid wide, short sleeves that will make your arms look big). The hem should sit at your hip bone (but be careful it isn't too wide here, or it will make you look wide). If you've got large breasts or a short neck, a lengthening V-neckline will be the most flattering (be careful you don't show too much cleavage). If you've got love handles or a big tummy, go for non-clinging cotton in a straight-cut style.

The crisp cotton shirt is a wardrobe 'must' for the older woman. There's nothing quite like its light-reflecting properties for flattering your complexion. It makes you look fresh and effortlessly stylish. It can be worn with jeans, trousers and skirts. It can go out to dinner, or on a weekend sailing trip. It says class and style with echoes of Grace Kelly and Katharine Hepburn.

The white shirt

The classic men's style can look great on a bigger, taller woman. A style that is slightly fitted is ideal for the curvier woman. The perfect fit is wide enough on the shoulders but not pulling across the chest. With shirts, you get what you pay for: the cut, fabric and whiteness are all better in a good-quality item.

In or out?

If you're big around the middle it's more flattering to let your shirt hang out – and a shaped, rather than straight, hem is the way to go. Otherwise, to wear it tucked in or left out is down to personal choice (and the appropriateness of the occasion).

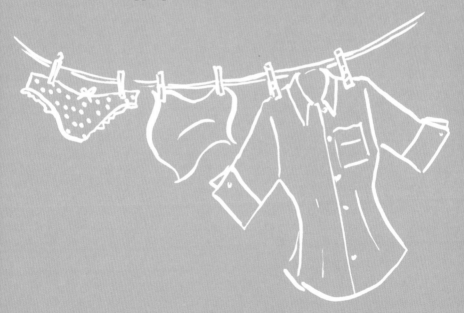

Dresses (for your shape)

The ease, simplicity and femininity of a dress is so alluring to the wearer. There are, however, a few rules. During the day, stick with the knee-skimming hemline. Shifts and A-lines beautifully hide a bit of a tummy, while a wrap (or cross-over) dress is great for women with curvy figures or big boobs. If you're worried about flabby or wrinkly arms, a good way to disguise them is with sheer sleeves or sleeves that end just before your elbow.

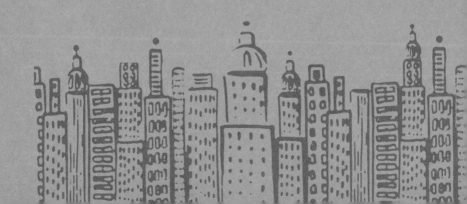

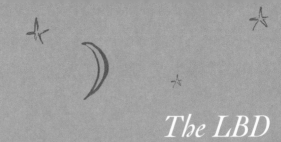

The LBD

Chic, uncomplicated and oh-so classy – the Little Black Dress is an essential item whatever your age. The funny thing about basic black is that it's not actually so basic; there are many versions of it, and the quality of the dress you buy will illustrate this. Cheap fabrics will have a slight blue or red tinge to them (if you've ever tried to co-ordinate a head-to-toe black outfit, you may have already come across this problem). Invest in a designer dress and you'll be rewarded with a great cut (which will hold its shape *forever*), great fabric (cotton, wool, silk, linen) and a brilliant fit (it will magically make you look 5kg lighter, and 5cm taller). You'll know it when you meet it, and it's worth every cent.

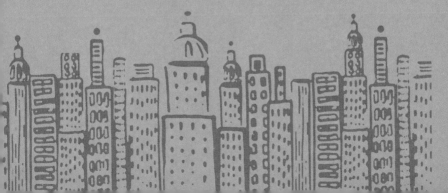

Skirt length and shape

Wear your skirts so they skim just under the knee – it's widely accepted as the most flattering length (hems that hit your calves at their widest point can make even the most elegant legs look short and stumpy). Wear long skirts with caution as they're hard to pull off if you're on the shorter side. A-line skirts flatter just about any shape because they skim the hips and slightly flare. Pencil skirts can look very elegant and sexy, if you've got the hips and rear end to carry it off.

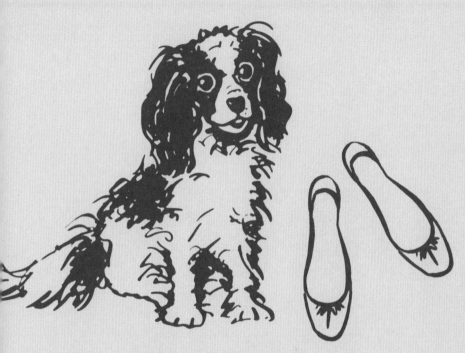

But which shoes?

Don't wear a long skirt with high heels (unless
you're thinking seriously formal evening-wear),
and definitely don't wear a long skirt with clumpy
shoes. Wear something simple such as ballet flats.

The *genius* of jeans

On paper it's simple: darker colours are more slimming; the classic boot-cut suits almost all shapes. That's in theory. In reality, you'll have to try on what seems like hundreds of pairs with what seems like the smallest of variations in fabric and cut before you hit the jackpot.

The perfect pair

Once you've found the perfect pair of jeans, buy champagne. And then go back and buy another pair. Finding the right jeans can take up a lot of shopping hours, but once you do, you'll wonder how you ever lived without them.

CONSIDER THIS . . .

★ If you are on the larger side, don't head straight for baggy jeans. They can make you look bigger than you are.

★ Elasticised waists and jeans with detailing (lace, studs, etc) are never cool.

★ Check how the fly sits: zips can be less bulky than buttons.

★ A high waistline accentuates the length of your hips and bum – and sadly only serves to make the whole area look larger.

★ Jeans with a slight stretch are infinitely more comfortable and figure-flattering.

★ If you aren't tall, skinny and 16 be wary of jeans with slim-fit legs.

★ The boot-cut gives the most slimming, lengthening look.

★ The most flattering waistline is just under your natural waist (don't go too low or too high).

★ Boot-cut jeans worn with heeled boots will make your legs look longer.

★ Believe it or not, bigger back pockets can make your bum look smaller.

Plus-size style

If you are not as slim as you used to be, there
are a few visual tricks that can help:

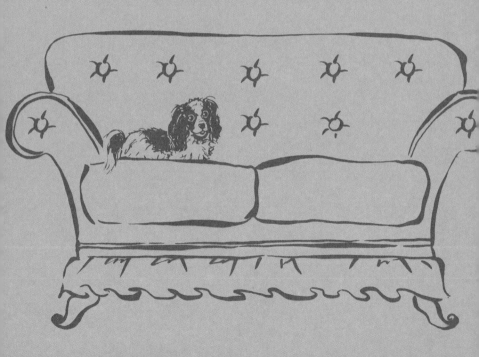

Keep it simple – monochrome basics
are eternally slimming.

✱

Wear shapes that skim your figure – avoid the tent
or tube look at all costs.

✱

Clever layering is the larger person's best friend
(watch out for bulkiness).

✱

Distract the eye with beautiful (preferably vertically
dominant) accessories, such as a long rope of beads,
or dangling earrings.

✱

Emphasise your great points: buy fabulous heels if your
calves are beautiful; wear V-necks if you have a lovely
décolletage.

✱

Keep waistlines simple with as little fabric as possible.
Go for skirts and pants with side zips.

✱

Wear tops and shirts that skim the top of your hips
(make sure they don't finish at the widest part of you).

Shoes

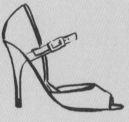

In your 60s, shoes are probably one of the most important clothing items you will buy. They must be stylish but comfortable – which means you should be prepared to invest in quality. As a rule of thumb, the softer the leather the more comfortable the shoe (never buy synthetic shoes). Look for non-slip rubber soles, or have new pairs re-soled for safety. Inner soles and arch support can greatly help – a qualified podiatrist can diagnose and address your requirements.

Bags

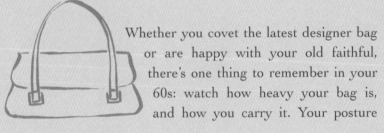

Whether you covet the latest designer bag or are happy with your old faithful, there's one thing to remember in your 60s: watch how heavy your bag is, and how you carry it. Your posture (and therefore health) can be affected if you carry your handbag on the same side every day. Remember to alternate sides, keep an eye on whether you're stooping, and regularly de-clutter your bag so it's lighter.

Baubles

Jewellery says a lot about a person. Even if you are on a budget you can make the most of the clothes you have by adding classic pearls and silver, or chunky ethnic pieces. It's your choice, your expression of style. There is infinite pleasure to be had trawling through accessories shops and antique markets for delicious accessories. Treasure your special pieces, and have fun with costume jewellery and the trends that come and go. Worn with discretion, jewellery can make an outfit. It's worth noting the sage advice to check your outfit in the mirror before you walk out the door – and remove one piece of jewellery.

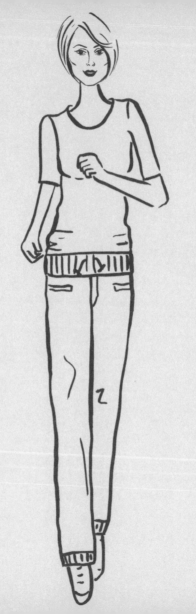

Body

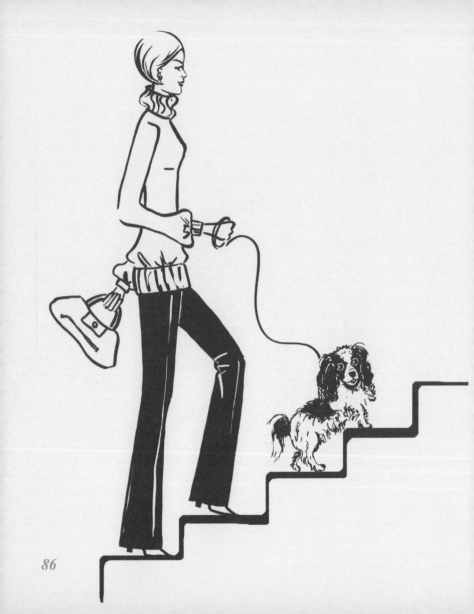

*T*his is your chance to really set yourself up for the coming decades. It's never too late to begin eating well and exercising regularly, but the sooner you start, the better off you'll be. Particular issues to watch out for are: dehydration (many of us are chronically dehydrated); a varied diet (your meals need to be as fresh and colourful as possible); bone loss (osteoporosis can be helped with diet and exercise); and a general lack of strength and flexibility. You don't have to make massive changes today. Every little bit counts. Enlist the help of your girlfriends in setting and sticking to goals, and encourage each other to work on your diet and exercise regimen – every day.

Food as medicine

Don't automatically presume that, just because you are 60-plus, you need to start popping pills. Use food as you would medicine – a visit to a naturopath or dietician will identify areas for improvement in your day-to-day diet. The best thing you can do for yourself is to eat a variety of fresh foods every day, as unprocessed as possible (and organic if you can afford it). A healthy diet is, quite simply, going to go a long way in keeping the doctor away.

Tea, ladies?

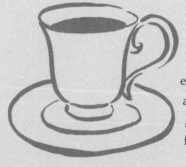

Drinking three or four cups of tea a day can cut down the risk of heart disease, stroke and cancer. It can even be beneficial for your bones, and help prevent dental plaque and gum disease. What are you waiting for? Put the kettle on.

A SAMPLE DIET

Breakfast
*a bowl of porridge (oatmeal) with natural yoghurt,
honey and dark berries or a poached egg on grain toast*

Morning tea
a handful of almonds and dried fruit

Lunch
*a mixed green salad with low-fat cheese or tuna, and
grain bread, or minestrone soup with a wholemeal roll*

Afternoon tea
low-fat yoghurt

Dinner
*grilled salmon with steamed vegetables and baby
potatoes or a lean-beef stir-fry with crisp green
vegetables served with brown rice*

It matters where you carry fat

Carrying weight around your stomach and back is far more harmful than having hip and thigh fat. Abdominal fat is more 'active' and, by releasing more fatty acids, can lead to heart disease and hardening of the arteries. Have your GP measure your waist and hips, to see if you sit in the safe zone.

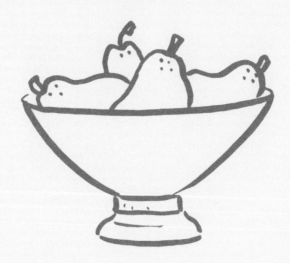

It's good to know your Body Mass Index. This is the measurement that gives a rough guide of whether you are overweight, underweight or in the healthy weight range. If you aren't a maths whizz, you'll find that quite a few of the bigger pharmacies (and, of course, your GP) will measure it for you. Otherwise, divide your weight in kilograms by your height in metres squared (for example, if you weigh 60kg and are 1.7m tall, your BMI will be 60 divided by 2.9, which is about 20.5).

What's your BMI?

Underweight = less than 18.5

Normal weight = 18.5–24.9

Overweight = 25–29.9

Obese = 30 or greater

Don't be fooled by food labels

Make sure you take your strongest glasses to the supermarket and properly examine the food labels, which are invariably in Lilliputian-size print:

No/low cholesterol or cholesterol free

This means exactly what it says: the product is low in cholesterol. What it does not mean is that it is healthy. It can be chock full of fat. The claims 'no cholesterol', 'low cholesterol' or 'cholesterol free' on products derived from plants, such as margarine and oil, are meaningless because all plant foods contain almost no cholesterol.

Reduced fat

This means the fat content is reduced from the original product. It should have been reduced by at least 25 per cent from the original. It does not necessarily mean that it is low in fat.

Low fat
The product must contain less than 3 per cent fat. Full cream milk is 4 per cent fat. Also beware: if an item claims to be 80 per cent fat free, it actually contains a whopping 20 per cent fat!

Fat free
These products must have less than 0.15 per cent fat.

Light or lite
These terms – even the misspelled ones – can refer to the appearance of the food (the texture or colour) and do not necessarily have anything to do with fat content. However, the characteristic that makes the food 'light' must be stated on the label.

No added sugar
This does not mean 'no sugar'.

Baked, not fried
You would think this means the product is low in fat and therefore healthier, but it can still have just as much fat. Check the nutrition panel to be sure.

Your bones are alive from birth to death, and their health depends on what you eat and how active you are. We need 1000 milligrams of calcium a day, but most women don't get nearly enough. Supplements can help slow the bone loss process but not stop it altogether. The best calcium-rich foods are dairy products, but be sure to stick to low-fat varieties as much as you can. Soy products can also help slow bone loss. Just one serve a day – soy milk, yoghurt, ice-cream or fortified bread – can make a difference.

Eating for strong bones

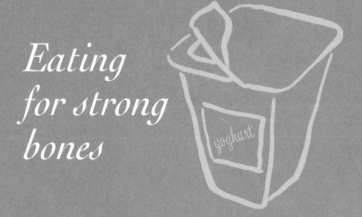

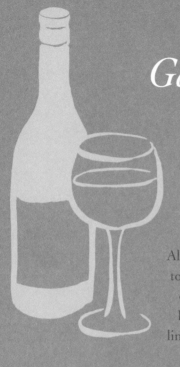

Good to know

Alcohol slows the body's ability to metabolise oestrogen, which can protect against bone loss. However, too much alcohol is linked to other health problems such as breast cancer. HRT (hormone replacement therapy) has also been shown to prevent bone loss, but some studies have linked it to heart attack and stroke in older, post-menopausal women.

Boning up on exercise

In your 60s, it's important to do exercise that stimulates bone building. Not all exercise does this: for example, swimming and bike riding are good for heart health, but don't build bones. The best ones are 'weight bearing' and make your body work against gravity. Running, brisk walking, stair climbing, dancing, skipping, tennis and netball are all good options. Each time your foot hits the ground you apply stress to your bones; the higher the impact, the greater the benefit to your bones. When it comes to strengthening bones in your hands, wrists, arms and shoulders, try boxing.

Here's an idea

It is important to see your doctor and have a bone-density test done. If needed, there are osteoporosis medications available.

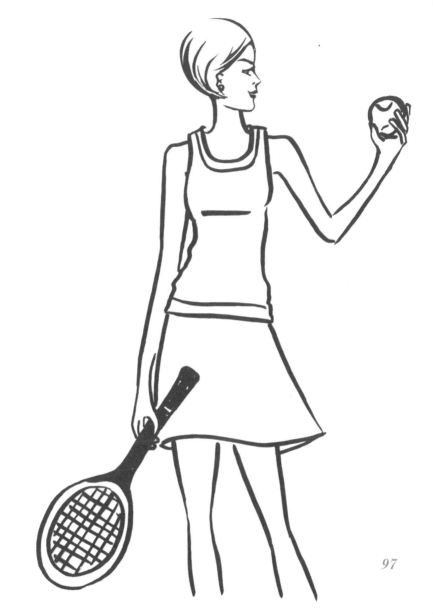

From our early 30s we lose about 1 per cent of muscle mass every year; by your 60s you will probably have lost about 30 per cent. But why is this important? The more muscle we have, the stronger we are, and this is vital for balance and the prevention of osteoporosis. But muscle has another role to play. It governs our metabolism. Put simply, the more muscle we have, the higher our metabolic rate. And the higher our metabolic rate, the easier it is to stay slim. So make sure your exercise regimen includes some weight training. The good news is that, even if you have already lost quite a bit of muscle, it's never too late to start building it up again.

Muscle up to stay slim

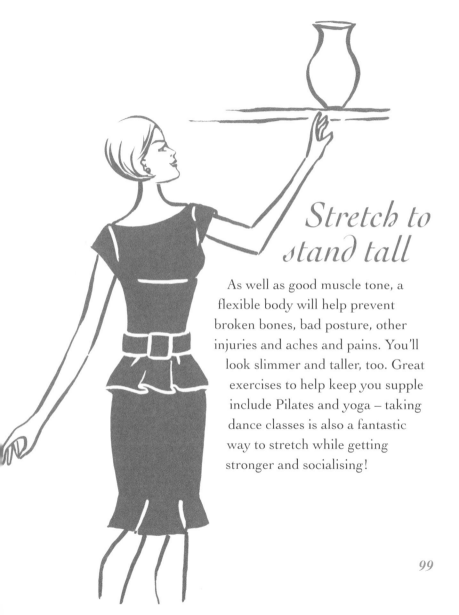

Stretch to stand tall

As well as good muscle tone, a flexible body will help prevent broken bones, bad posture, other injuries and aches and pains. You'll look slimmer and taller, too. Great exercises to help keep you supple include Pilates and yoga – taking dance classes is also a fantastic way to stretch while getting stronger and socialising!

Did you know that about half of all women over 60 have trouble rising from a chair? If you can't get up from sitting without using your hands, you need to develop your leg strength. Walking, cycling and swimming will help, as will specific weight-training exercises at a gym.

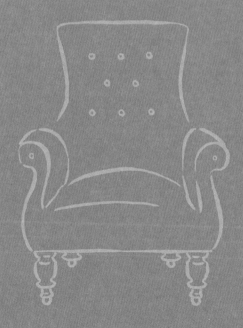

DIY LEG EXERCISE

1 *Stand behind a chair with both hands on the back of the chair to help you balance.*

2 *Position your feet about shoulder-width apart.*

3 *Pretend to sit down by flexing your knees and sticking out your bottom.*

4 *Only go down as far as it feels comfortable and then slowly rise up again.*

Do about 10 squats at a time (as you get stronger it will get easier).

The best exercise for you

**If you want to be fit and healthy in your 60s,
the optimal exercise program involves *variety*:**

Walk whenever possible

✱

Do exercise that improves and maintains balance

✱

Stretch regularly

✱

Do cardio, such as a slow jog, three days a week

✱

Weight train, using light weights, three days a week

Moderation is key

Only take any exercise to the level at which you feel comfortable. Be careful with exercises that over-stress your joints. But moderate aches and pains shouldn't be an excuse to do no exercise at all. Declining cardio fitness, strength and flexibility is not the inevitable consequence of ageing. It's due to lack of use.

Best non-jarring exercises

Yoga   Pilates   Tai chi   Swimming   Aqua-aerobics

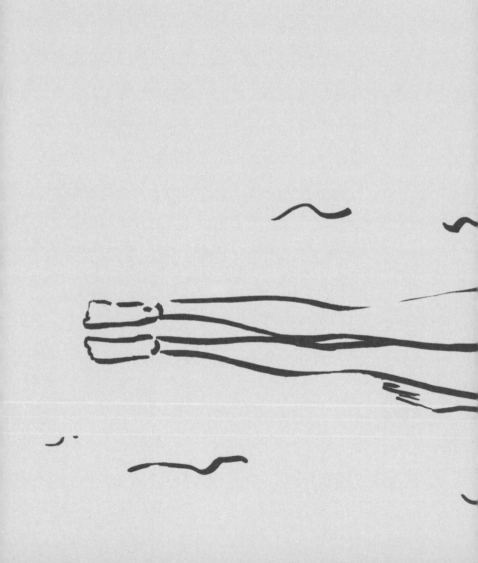

Health

You're a long time alive

Think about this: in 1900 when Australia first introduced the aged pension for people aged 65 and over, the average lifespan was just 62. Now, a woman who turned 50 in 2003 can expect to live beyond 100. Through better nutrition and huge advances in medicine and healthcare, we're all living longer. The goal these days is not only to live longer, but to be healthier while we're doing it.

Food for thought

Just like the rest of your body, your brain needs feeding. It is fuelled by glucose but that doesn't mean you should live on a diet of sugar – quite the reverse. Research has shown that a low-GI, high-fibre diet works best, and you particularly need the following nutrients:

* Omega-3 fatty acids or DHA. Fish that contains DHA is the best brain food. Not only will it feed and lubricate the brain, DHA is thought to help stave off dementia and Alzheimer's.

* Antioxidants (beta-carotene and vitamins C and E). These mop up damaging free radicals that circulate throughout the body.

* Vitamin B. An Australian study found that a diet rich in B vitamins improves your capacity to think and remember.

* Plus, don't eat junk food. Food that contains trans-fats has been shown to accelerate brain cell loss.

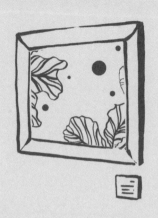
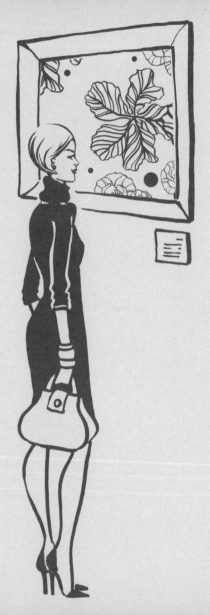

Cigarettes and your brain

Despite a scattering of media stories claiming that smoking helps to prevent Alzheimer's Disease because nicotine can temporarily improve brain function, the overwhelming opinion is that smoking constricts and damages blood vessels and is more likely to cause brain impairment. It is certainly a factor in causing stroke.

Get out and about

People who have an active social life are less likely to suffer memory problems as they get older. If your partner complains that you do all the talking, just tell them that you are exercising your brain.

If you stay awake for 21 hours straight, your thinking and problem-solving abilities are equivalent to someone who is legally drunk. Sleep is when your brain processes new memories, hones new skills and solves problems. Have you ever found that when trying to learn something new, things seemed much clearer the next day? This is because while you are asleep your brain reactivates the circuits it was using as you learned, rehearses them, and then moves the new memories into long-term storage. There is also some evidence that sleep can help produce moments of problem-solving insight. Complex things that seemed confusing one day can suddenly make sense the next.

Get a good night's sleep

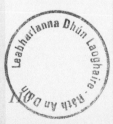

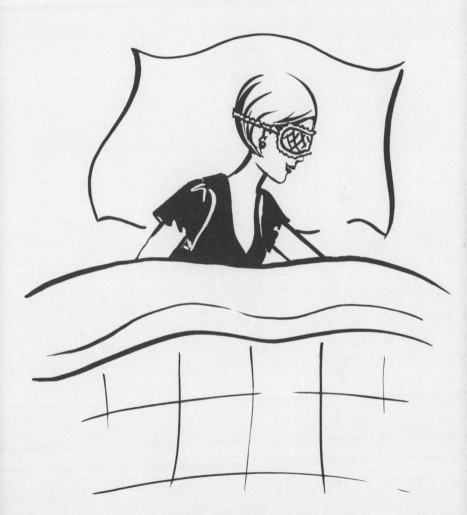

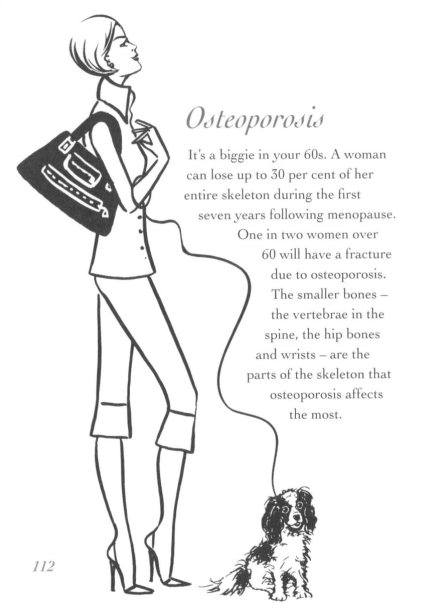

Osteoporosis

It's a biggie in your 60s. A woman
can lose up to 30 per cent of her
entire skeleton during the first
seven years following menopause.
One in two women over
60 will have a fracture
due to osteoporosis.
The smaller bones –
the vertebrae in the
spine, the hip bones
and wrists – are the
parts of the skeleton that
osteoporosis affects
the most.

We're all aware of the dangers of the sun's UV rays in causing skin cancer and accelerating skin ageing. The trouble is, you need UV rays to make vitamin D – an important must-have for post-menopausal women because it helps your body absorb calcium and repair bones. You make vitamin D when the UV rays in sunlight hit your skin, and 10 minutes of sun exposure a day is sufficient. To get enough vitamin D from diet alone, you would have to drink 10 big glasses of fortified milk every day.

Here comes the sun

Dicky knees

Snap, crackle, pop . . . Yep, it's those knees
again. If you stop to think about how much
work they do every day, it's no surprise they protest.
Here are some facts:

* Women suffer more than men (due to our wider pelvises).

* As we age, we lose muscle – 1 per cent a year from
our 30s – which puts more strain on the knee joint.

* Post-menopausal bone loss affects our knees.

* Carrying extra weight adds more stress on knee joints.

* Bad posture is a big contributor.

* High heels make things worse, as do shoes
that make you walk flat-footed.

So, what to do

- ✱ Improve your posture.

- ✱ Keep your weight down.

- ✱ Eat a calcium-rich diet.

- ✱ Do strengthening exercises – walking, weights, squats and lunges.

- ✱ Train your core muscles with yoga or Pilates.

- ✱ Stay supple – always warm up before and stretch after exercise.

- ✱ Use knee pads for housework and gardening.

- ✱ Watch your footwear and make sure you have arch support in your shoes.

- ✱ Listen to your knees. If the pain is really bad, see your doctor.

Ovarian cancer

The risk of ovarian cancer increases with age; the median age of diagnosis is 64 years. Each year about 1200 women are diagnosed in Australia and about 800 will die. This is because more than 70 per cent are diagnosed at an advanced stage, when the cancer has spread and is very difficult to treat successfully. Rates of survival are improving thanks to better treatment. The five-year survival rate for Australian women is now about 43 per cent compared with 34 per cent in the 1980s. Known risks include obesity, having a first child when you are over 30, fertility treatment and close family history.

Know your body

A new test for ovarian cancer has just been announced and will soon be available. In the meantime, the best thing you can do is to be aware of the (unfortunately very vague) symptoms and, if you notice any changes to your body, see your GP. Look out for:

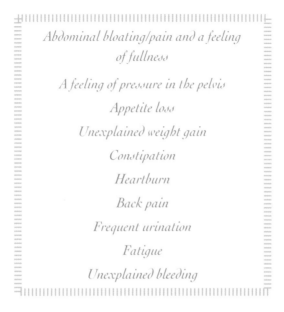

Abdominal bloating/pain and a feeling
of fullness

A feeling of pressure in the pelvis

Appetite loss

Unexplained weight gain

Constipation

Heartburn

Back pain

Frequent urination

Fatigue

Unexplained bleeding

Ovarian cancer and diet

A big US study of 50,000 women, published by the National Cancer Institute, showed that a low-fat diet (20 per cent of overall diet, along with plenty of fruit, vegetables and wholegrains) may lower the risk of ovarian cancer in post-menopausal women.

Brushing may save your life

A recent survey found the rate of gum disease has almost doubled among the over-60s in Australian in the past 14 years. The problem is that gum disease has been linked with an increased risk of heart attack, stroke, diabetes and osteoporosis. One theory is that oral bacteria can affect the heart when it enters the bloodstream. So brush twice a day and don't forget to floss.

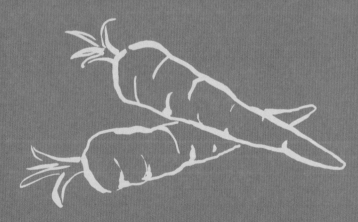

You can now have a blood test that will help you live as long as possible. A world-first test developed by Adelaide doctors and the CSIRO can identify your level of DNA damage and the nutrient levels in your blood. The Genome Health Analysis is aimed at helping you make lifestyle and medical decisions to maximise your chance of living a long and healthy life. The test looks for specific DNA damage that can flag future ailments, as well as the nutrient levels in your blood.

Happy century

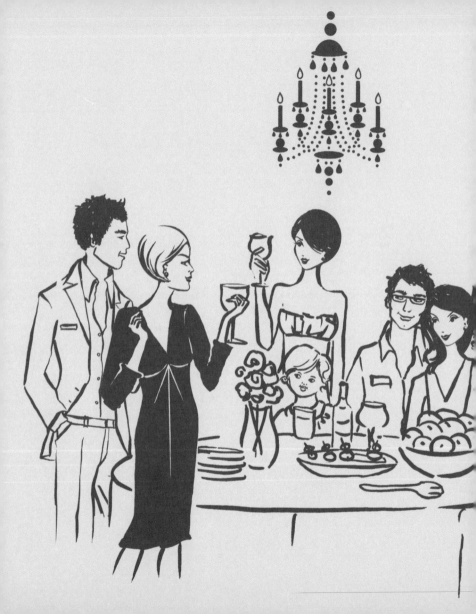

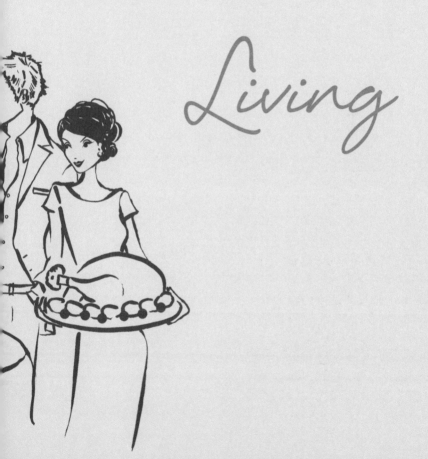

Living

Retirement?

It's one of the biggest life changes we face. We daydream that we'll travel, buy a B&B, write that novel, sail around the world, live near the kids, move away from the kids . . . But as it gets closer, nothing is as easy as it seemed. The prospect of decades ahead with little to do while eking out your superannuation is, not surprisingly, a hard thing for the modern-day woman to swallow. This dilemma is a recent phenomenon. Our parents and grandparents were not blessed with such longevity or the choice to stop working at 65. View this exciting time as the perfect chance to make a real contribution to society, and work on those personal changes you've been dying to address.

Ageing is in your head

That's the collective message from a whole range of research scientists. We once thought that the body and the brain packed it in soon after retirement but we now know better. Through diet and exercise we can stay physically healthy, but it's the way we approach life that makes the real difference.

A woman's best friend

With a little more time on your hands, your 60s is the perfect time to enjoy the delights of pet ownership.

Having a pet can be one of life's greatest privileges and the deep connection we have with our furry little mates can be both humbling and inspiring. They give us unconditional love and see us through troubled times. They can be a best friend, a confidant, and let's be honest – most of us regard our pets as one of the family.

There are plenty of studies showing the benefits of pet ownership. One big Australian project showed pet owners had lower blood pressure and lower cholesterol levels than non pet owners. Other research has found that pets can help people recuperate after serious illness and give people a better chance of recovering from a heart attack.

In your 60s you can often give a pet more time. Dogs especially hate being alone and even 'the cat who walks by herself' actually prefers company.

But be careful: too many pets are bought on impulse, turn out to be unsuitable and are dumped at shelters. Make sure you find the right pet for your lifestyle. Whether you go for a cat or dog, check out lists of breeds, their personality types and the environment they thrive in. Think about your home and the people in it: do you want a devoted one-woman pet or a life-of-the-party animal? If you're not stuck on best of breed, consider a rescue cat or dog. Moggies and mongrels can be just as endearing as a purebred and you'll probably be saving a life.

Living with and enjoying a close relationship with our pets can be one of life's sublime pleasures. If it's something you've longed to do – go for it. You'll never regret it.

Keep busy

The latest research says you'll be happier, healthier and wealthier if you decide to keep on working at something that matters to you. If your present job is less than satisfying, you should consider a career change (yes, it can be done in your 60s!). Importantly, it has been shown that people who stay active maintain social networks and are fitter than those who don't – both vital to a healthy old age.

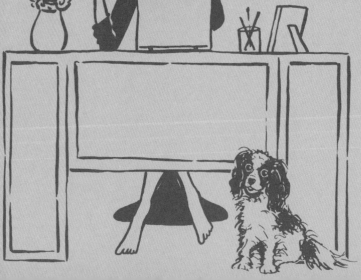

THE CHECKLIST

The idea is to identify what matters most to you
in the second half of life and plan accordingly.
Consider:

Working part time

Setting up a business from home

Developing a hobby into a business

Becoming involved in your community

Helping family members and friends

Learning a new skill

Taking up a new sport or activity

Volunteering for a charity organisation,
either at home or overseas

Now, where did I leave them?

As we get older, we all worry about our memory; every time we forget where we've put the car keys, a little voice whispers: Alzheimer's . . . But don't panic: Alzheimer's does affect some people, but only about 1 per cent of people in their 60s. The reality is that young people forget things too – it just doesn't bother them. The results from a number of recent studies suggest that most of us maintain excellent memory and brain function right into old age.

It's on the tip of my tongue...

This phenomenon – when your mind freezes when you're searching for a crucial word, such as someone's name – happens to everybody. It is more likely to occur if it's a word you haven't spoken aloud for some time. This is because you are actually having trouble retrieving the sound of the word from your memory. Some brain functions get better with age. Research has shown that older people are better at judging a person's character.

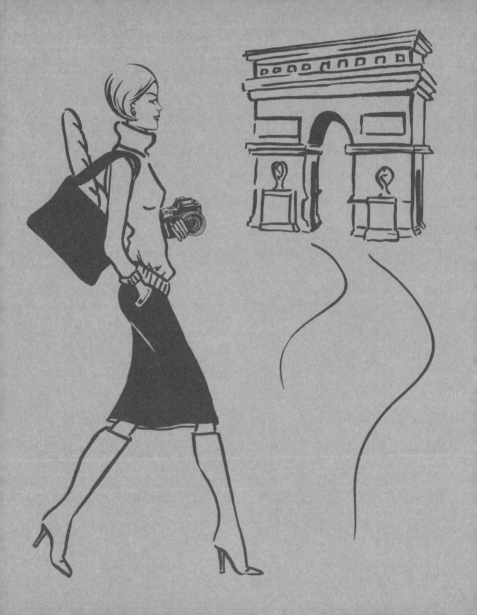

Run your way to a better brain

Research is showing that exercise can help stimulate neurogenesis, your brain's regeneration process. The birth of new brain cells is our body's way of adapting to environmental changes, and it plays an important role in learning and memory. Studies have shown that even a short jog can make all the difference, and scientists are researching the theory that exercise can stave off Alzheimer's disease.

Or learn French . . .

Memory is like everything else in the body – use it or lose it. You can slow mental ageing by exercising your brain. Stretching yourself, through learning something new, is a great brain workout. Learn a language, or how to play the piano or chess, or complete cryptic crosswords.

Some ideas to get you going

The UK's University of Southampton recommends the following brain 'exercises':

* Get involved in something that requires mental activity: crosswords, Sudoku, reading, evening classes, card games or discussion groups.

* When you are reading a good book or a newspaper article, pause every now and again and imagine you are telling someone about what you have just read.

* Form or join a book group to discuss what you're reading with other people.

* In the evening, try to recall the day's events in as much detail as possible.

* Have a debate with yourself. Pick a topic and think up some opinions opposite to those that you usually hold.

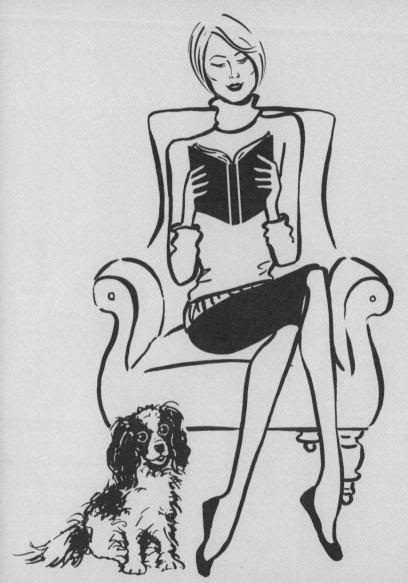

Volunteering

If you want to make a difference to the world, there are a number of organisations that are very keen to hear from you. Volunteers are needed locally and all over the world. A good place to start is www.volunteeringaustralia. org – the umbrella body for volunteers – and then go to www.govolunteer.com for a list of organisations and their profiles. There is evidence to show that volunteering, whether for two weeks or two years, is a life-enriching experience.

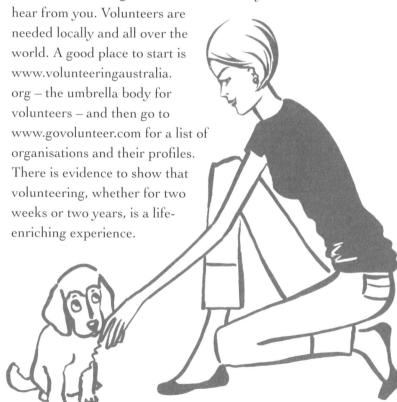

Ask yourself what you want to gain from the experience. Apart from helping others, is it about living in another country, expanding your social networks with like-minded people, getting away from the daily grind? Are you interested in children, animals, women's health or the underprivileged? Consider your personality and be truthful with yourself. Can you get along with a range of different people from different social and cultural backgrounds?

Which charity to choose?

What do you have to offer?

You don't have to be a nurse, social worker or teacher to make a difference. Your lifetime of experience can be put to use in many ways. There are many local or smaller projects that simply need an extra pair of hands. At the other end of the scale, larger projects need specific skills and training – people with financial, technical or management experience.

Volunteering overseas

This is a big undertaking – but one that is a lifelong dream for many, and extremely enriching. The websites mentioned previously will point you in the right direction. You will need to be physically and emotionally resilient. Most overseas projects will expect you to pay for your own travel expenses, although some will help with accommodation and food. Plan your finances wisely and don't forget insurance.

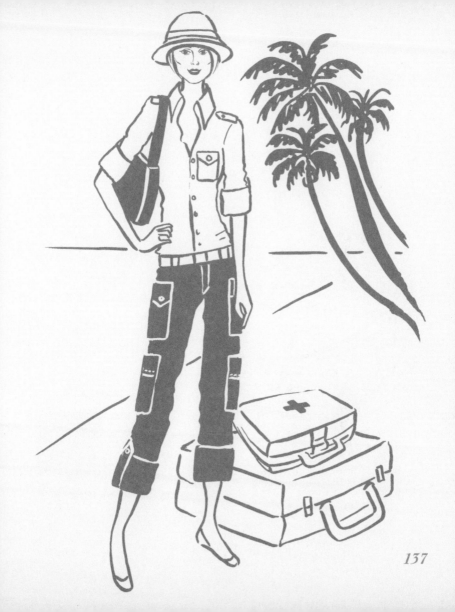

The world is your oyster

For some, the 60s is when all the hard work you have done over many decades is finally reaping rewards: if you have kids they've flown the nest, you might be able to spend less time at work and, if you're lucky, there's a little bit of money to spend on yourself. All that means one thing: this is the perfect time to travel.

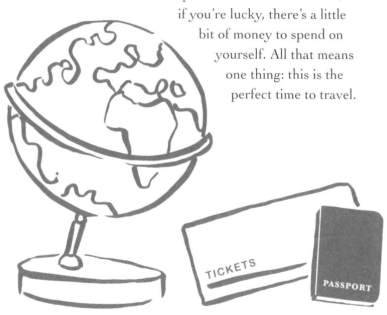

From taking a campervan around Australia to cruising through the Greek Islands on board a yacht, there is a trip to suit your taste and style. If archaeology is your thing, why not try Egypt? But don't feel there's anything wrong with a shopping jaunt to Paris, London or New York, either! Take your partner or a friend with similar interests, or be brave and go by yourself – you never know who you will meet.

Pitter-patter

If your younger years were devoted to raising children, then by now you might have earned one or two of those wonderful creatures, grandchildren. Whether you look after them on a regular basis one or two days a week or you just see them on special occasions, you'll get to enjoy all the bliss of little children again – with the added bonus that you can give them back when they get tired and cranky. Truly the best of both worlds!

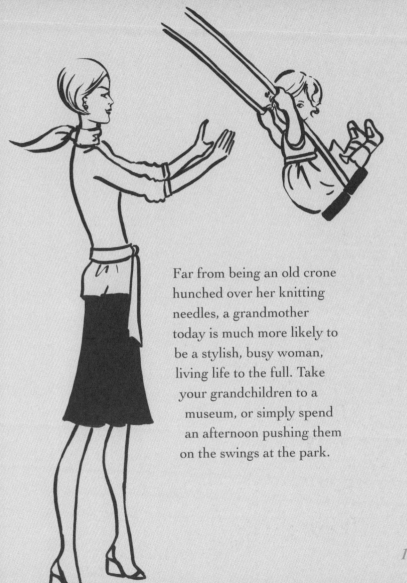

Far from being an old crone
hunched over her knitting
needles, a grandmother
today is much more likely to
be a stylish, busy woman,
living life to the full. Take
your grandchildren to a
museum, or simply spend
an afternoon pushing them
on the swings at the park.

There's a saying that goes: 'Have something to do, someone to love and something to look forward to.' Keeping busy, working on your relationships and dreaming big dreams is the *real* fountain of youth!

Anti-ageing secret:
don't stop working or learning

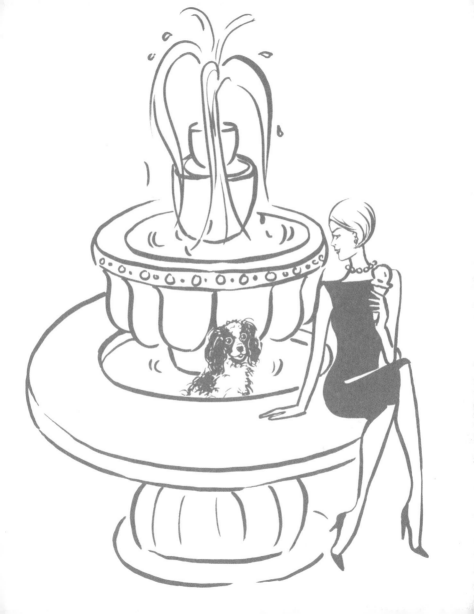

An Ebury Press book
Published by Random House Australia Pty Ltd
Level 3, 100 Pacific Highway, North Sydney, NSW 2060
www.randomhouse.com.au

First published by Ebury Press in 2008

Addresses for companies within the Random House Group can be found at
www.randomhouse.com.au/offices.

National Library of Australia
Cataloguing-in-Publication Entry

Robson, Pamela.
Grown-up & gorgeous in your 60s.

ISBN 978 1 74166 803 2 (pbk.)

Beauty, Personal.
Women – Health and hygiene.
Older women – Health and hygiene.

646.7042

Cover and internal illustrations by Megan Hess
Cover design by Christabella Designs
Internal design by Anna Warren, Warren Ventures Pty Ltd
Additional design by Liz Seymour, Seymour Designs
Printed and bound by Tien Wah Press (PTE), Singapore

Random House Australia uses papers that are natural, renewable and recyclable products and made
from wood grown in sustainable forests. The logging and manufacturing processes are expected to
conform to the environmental regulations of the country of origin.

10 9 8 7 6 5 4 3 2 1